W9-COS-632

RISK

Rachel MacKenzie

RISK

New York   The Viking Press

RISK

✤

For Gennie and Ruth

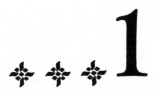

"I THINK IT'S TIME YOU SAW A SUPER-SUPER HEART man," Dr. Lewis said. "You remember, I told you I might want you to. We'll make the arrangements and be in touch."

The appointment with Dr. Jamison was for January 13. "I have your September hospital record," he said when she called from the office where she worked, "and I've talked with Dr. Lewis and have his recent cardiograms and X-ray. I guess that's everything I need."

"Except me," she said.

"Well, yes," Dr. Jamison said after a slight pause.

Now he perched himself on the desk in the hospital examining room and looked down on her. "Has Dr. Lewis talked to you about your situation?"

"Not as much as I'd like."

"Well, I'm going to. When I've spent this much time with a patient, I feel I should tell her what I think. It's congestive heart failure, as you already know. There's fluid. You have a murmur—two on a scale of six, not too bad. What I want to do is this: shift your medication around a bit"—he explained —"and if you aren't considerably better in six to eight weeks, then I feel we should do a much more intensive examination

3

to consider the possibility of surgery. After all, you're a comparatively young woman."

It was such a shock she said nothing. She held her face very still.

"Heart X-rays," he said.

"More than the X-rays I've already had? I work, you know. Is it something I could come in and have done in a day?"

"No, no. You'd have to be *in* the hospital for them—I'd say a week to ten days. Count on ten days. There are two: a heart catheterization and an arteriogram. We'd have to get you ready, and then you'd need three or four days to recover from the first before we did the second, and a few days to recover from that. They're quite different from anything you've had. They're done with dye and give us a look inside the heart, inside the coronary artery."

"Is there any risk?" she asked.

"There's always risk in a procedure that involves the heart. But if anything goes wrong you're with people who know exactly what to do and have the equipment to do it with. They're prepared." He smiled. He was a tall, handsome man, not personal but kindly, and everything he said was very clear. They had just spent two hours together.

"Why do I have to wait?" she asked.

"I want to try you on this change of medication," he said. "You might not have to have them done." He smiled again.

"Are you a surgeon?"

"No, I don't do surgery."

"I love being alive," she said inconsequentially.

●   ●   ●

"What exactly are those X-rays?" she asked Dr. Lewis when

she saw him three days later. She'd known him longer, though not long, really—only a few months—but she found it easier to put her questions to him. Besides, it took time for her to find her questions. They always came late. Her mind turned things over, and there they were.

"A heart catheterization and an arteriogram, I would suppose. Didn't Dr. Jamison tell you?"

"Yes, and he explained them some, but I stopped listening. Taking it in, anyway. They run a catheter into your heart?"

"Yes," he said. "And take X-rays. It's quite dramatic. Lots of people around. You're in a big dark room, with an enormous light over you."

"Does Dr. Jamison do them?"

"No. It's a highly specialized department. Dr. Allen."

"Why do I have to wait?" she said. "Waiting is the hardest."

He was as cross as he got with her. "The tests would be meaningless in the shape you're in now. We have to get you in optimum shape for them to make sense."

"I mind waiting," she said.

Two days later, Dr. Lewis called her at home. "I've been talking to Dr. Jamison," he said. "We've made a reservation for you for February twenty-second. We tried to set one up earlier, but the schedule was full the week we wanted, and then Dr. Jamison will be off for ten days, skiing. It's important that he be here. February twenty-second is the first date we could arrange. I'm sorry. That's a Sunday. The catheterization will be done on Wednesday."

"Wednesday!" she said.

"It takes some preparation," he said. "And we want you rested."

That evening she hung a large calendar on the wall at the foot of her bed and circled Sunday, February 22, and Wednesday, February 25. It was the first that any of this seemed real.

Another question had turned up, and the next time she was in Dr. Lewis's office she said diffidently, "Suppose they find surgery *is* possible, is there any chance that they'll move straight into it? I would need to do something about the office if there is—say something. . . ."

He looked at her thoughtfully. "Yes," he said. "Or we might let you out for two weeks if there were personal things you had to attend to."

Another shock.

"Where would the incision be?"

He was sitting at his desk, and he reached over and very lightly traced a line down the middle of her chest, curving toward the left, low under her breast. "Here, I would think." His expression was fastidious.

She shivered, but not so that it could be seen. "Do you think it's going to be possible?"

"We have to wait for the results of the tests. But remember, if it isn't, I can help you." He smiled. He had a lovely smile, warm and encompassing.

Help me adjust to a life in bed, she thought. Still, she smiled back.

The weeks were slow. "Where do you suppose they run the catheter *from*?" she asked Ellie, who lived with her—an adopted sister.

"I haven't the faintest idea."

"The bend of the arm is my guess."

"No, I think the wrist—or maybe it's the shoulder. I think maybe I've heard that."

"But how could they possibly get into a *shoulder?*"

For some reason, she was shy about asking Dr. Lewis, even though it was the question they discussed most at home. Well, what else was there? To the people she worked with she said only that she had to go into the hospital for a week to ten days for some tests. They all knew she was in trouble, and how could you announce you were going to have something before you knew you were going to have it? But she made a new will, she took care of her income taxes, she transferred money to her checking account and executed a power of attorney for Ellie to be able to draw on it. She got as much work in the office done ahead as she could, and papers at home put in order. And the waiting seemed to go on forever.

• • •

When they went to the hospital, she was having difficulty with her breathing. A woman from the admitting office came out to the waiting room with papers for her to sign, and a few minutes later brought the plastic identification band to fasten around her wrist; they hardly had to wait at all. And then they were upstairs in a tiny dark box of a room, and the nurses took over.

In the late afternoon, when Ellie was off buying a plant to cheer the place up, a nurse came in. She had a large red book under her arm, and she sat down by the bed and held it open on her lap. "I've come to prepare you for your heart catheterization," she announced.

There didn't seem anything to say to that.

The nurse consulted her book. "This is a procedure by

which catheters are introduced into the heart and X-rays are taken."

"Catheters? More than one?"

The nurse looked down at her book. "Yes. Two."

"Can you tell me where they're inserted?"

The nurse consulted the book again. "I'm afraid I don't know. It isn't a procedure I'm familiar with, myself. Your doctor can tell you. Yours is scheduled for Wednesday morning. Someone will come down from the department to go over it all with you. No breakfast that morning. Nothing by mouth after midnight—the usual."

"Does that mean it's done under anesthesia?"

Another look at the book. "I really couldn't tell you. You'll have to ask your doctor."

"Is the catheterization done under anesthesia?" she asked Dr. Lewis when he came in for a visit in the early evening.

"No," he said. "Just a sedative. They have to have your co-operation for the X-rays."

"I've been prepared out of a big red book," she said, "but it didn't seem to have all the answers."

They laughed together.

"I have a horror of anesthesia," she said.

"I want to prepare you for your heart catheterization," Dr. Jamison said Monday morning after he'd examined her. He was wonderfully tanned from his ten days of skiing. "It's a little rugged. They run two catheters into the heart—one through a vein in here"—he touched the bend of her right arm—"and one through the femoral artery. It's marvelous what the X-rays show us; they're a marvelous diagnostic aid.

The whole thing should take three, maybe three and a half hours. It may bother your back, having to lie in one position so long. They use a dye for the last pictures. Some people have a reaction to that, but there's no reason you should. We've stopped your anticoagulant and will be giving you some Vitamin K. Do you have any questions?"

"No," she said. "I guess they're all answered."

He tweaked her toe and was off.

"Hello. I'm Dr. Morris. I've come to prepare you for your heart catheterization," a very attractive young woman said on Tuesday afternoon. "I'll be in charge. The staff takes turns at it. Dr. Allen will do the X-rays at the end. Has anyone told you what to expect?"

"Well, I think so," she said.

"I'll go over it again. We use two catheters. We cut into a vein at the bend of your right arm for one, and use the right femoral artery for the other. They usually go in quite painlessly—not always. We use a little Novocain. Once they're in place, we manipulate them around the chambers and get a good many measurements—blood flow, volume, and so on— that are recorded on an electronic display. There's a constant cardiogram being taken. The X-rays are done at the end. If you're interested, you can watch part of it on the fluoroscopic screen. Some people can't stand to, and we turn the screen away from them, but some people like to see what's going on —it helps pass the time—and we're glad to let them. And to talk and explain things. It's just as you like. We talk among ourselves. It's quite informal."

"I'd like to watch," she said.

"Fine."

"Dr. Jamison said three to three and a half hours?"

"At the most," Dr. Morris said. "I should think less. Now if you'll just let me examine you . . ."

"If anything goes wrong," Dr. Jamison said on Tuesday after Dr. Morris's visit, "remember, you're with people who know what to do and have equipment."

"You mean a heart attack?"

"It's a possibility. I don't expect it. But if you have trouble you couldn't be in better hands."

Dr. Lewis came Tuesday evening. "All set?"

"I should think so."

"Oh, one thing. Don't be reluctant to tell Dr. Allen when you've had enough. He'll ask. I've explained to him that you have a bad back. It's a long time to be in one position, and that X-ray table is *hard*. I have clinic tomorrow, so I'll be dropping in on you."

• • •

There were five doctors in the room, all young, and out in the corridor a number of nurses. Two of them came in and moved her from the stretcher to the cold, hard table, and Dr. Morris introduced her around. The light overhead was enormous, and so was a rectangle at the foot of the table. It looked like a great fluorescent light. "What's that?" she asked.

"An electronic machine," Dr. Morris said. "It's keeps records—cardiogram and so on. You won't be able to see them; the blank side is toward you." The room was lined with equipment. A large construction back of her head was for the X-rays, they told her.

Two of the doctors covered her with sterile sheets. "Well, we might as well get to work," Dr. Morris said, and lifted her right arm. "I'm just going to cut into a vein. All you'll feel is the Novocain. Prick. We'll put a stitch in it at the end. We have a competition going to see who can come out with the smallest incision."

"Who's ahead?" she asked, terrified.

"It's a draw. Dr. Peterson here is pretty good. . . . *There* we are. By the way, be sure to let us know if at any time you have pain or feel odd in any way. I'm inserting the catheter."

"*That's* painful."

"Blast!" Dr. Morris said. "The vein's gone into spasm. I'm sorry, I'm going to have to hurt you."

She worked with the catheter for what seemed a very long time.

"The pain is quite bad."

"I know. Sometimes they slip through just like that. I'm going to have to get Dr. Allen," she said to the other young doctors gathered round.

"He won't thank you for interrupting him," one of them said.

"I can't help that—will you ask him to come in, please?"

"I'm Dr. Allen," he said to her. "I understand you're having some trouble." He took over the catheter. "I'm just going to have to force it through. Once we get past the axilla, we'll have smooth sailing. Oh, that axilla!"

The pain became excruciating.

"Hi." Dr. Lewis had come in. He spoke to Dr. Allen and

went to the head of the table and put his hands through the shelves there and placed them one on each side of her head. "Is it pretty bad?"

She nodded. "How much longer?"

"Not too long," Dr. Allen said. "We're almost there."

"You're doing all right," Dr. Lewis said. "I'll be back."

"There!" Dr. Allen said finally, and, sure enough, the pain had ended, though the word "excruciating" hung in her mind and wouldn't leave. "I'll see you later," he said to her, and to Dr. Morris, "Carry on. Let me know when you're ready."

"Now for the second," Dr. Morris said. "I'll just give you some Novocain. We have to push this one in—don't dare cut. It may hurt. Nothing like the other, though."

It hurt. There was a feeling of warmth running down her groin, and she thought they must be using warm water.

All the doctors were faced toward what looked like a television screen at her right. She turned her head to see, and there on the screen two long, thin, wormlike creatures moved in fluid in a vaguely chambered structure. Their movement was like a little dance. "Is that my *heart*?" she asked.

"That's right," one of the men said.

"But I never felt the second catheter except when you pushed it in. It was so fast."

"Will someone get Pat to come monitor the cardiogram?" Dr. Morris said, and to her, "Do you feel anything?"

"I'm aware they're there."

"But no pain? It's important that you let us know immediately if you have any pain in your chest." She began to manipulate the catheter in the arm; Dr. Peterson was manipulating the catheter in the groin. They were using warm water again.

"Try turning it to the right," Dr. Peterson said, and on the fluoroscope she saw one of the catheters dance. "You have it," he said, "You're in."

In what, she wondered.

Out of her sight a voice began in a monotone, "Beep . . . Beep . . . Beep, beep, beep . . . Beep . . . Beepbeepbeepbeep."

Dr. Lewis's hands were on her head again. She hadn't seen him come in. "All right?" he said. "Is your back hurting?"

"It's beginning to. I feel as if I'd been here a long time. What are those beeps?"

"Oh, they're just keeping track of the beat."

"Do you see my heart?"

"I see it. Everything looks fine. I've been over watching the cardiogram. I'll drop by," he said.

"Beep . . . Beep . . . Beepbeepbeep," the voice droned on. "Beepbeep."

Dr. Allen was at her side. "We're going to take the X-rays now," he said. "I'll just pull this machine over your chest. Don't worry, it won't crush you, though I do have to cut off your view. What we need from you is to lie perfectly still and hold your breath when I tell you."

It was a ponderous business, and it went on and on.

"I'm sorry, but I don't think I can stay in this position much longer," she said. "It's my back."

"Just five more minutes," Dr. Allen said. "Try moving that catheter—here, I'll do it." He came around to the side. *"Now* let's see what we get."

Plate after plate.

"I'm in too much pain to stand it any longer," she said half an hour later.

"Just five more minutes," Dr. Allen said from behind her head.

Dr. Lewis was there again. This time he stood at her side.

"My back's hurting," she told him.

"I'm not getting as clear pictures as I'd like," Dr. Allen said, and Dr. Lewis left to join him.

Then he was beside her once more. "I have to go keep office hours." He touched her lightly. "I'll be in to see you tonight. It shouldn't be much longer."

"Look, I really *can't* stand it," she said another half hour later. "If you'd just give me something to stop this pain in my back I'd be all right."

"We don't have anything of the sort up here," Dr. Allen said.

"Couldn't you get something?"

"Just five more minutes. We're ready to start the dye. It won't be long."

"You'll feel this the second we start," Dr. Peterson said. "Your mouth will dry up and you'll have a tingling sensation in your tongue and down your arms. Don't worry. It only makes a few people sick, but here's a basin, in case."

"Well, I guess that's the best I'm going to get," Dr. Allen said at last. "I'm sorry it took us so long." He shook her hand. "You were very patient." Three of the young doctors went out with him. Only Dr. Morris and Dr. Peterson were left.

"Maybe a pillow would help your back," Dr. Morris said. "We can't let you get up yet," and a nurse brought a pillow and wedged it under her left side. "We have to take the catheters out and put a stitch in your arm."

She bent her legs to shift the pressure on her back.

"Don't move that leg!" Dr. Peterson said sharply.

"Could I have a drink?"

"I don't see why not," he said, and he went out and brought her a tall glass of cold water with a curved straw.

"There!" Dr. Morris said when the stitch was in. "Now we'll get rid of the second one." She moved down the table.

"It's been more than three and a half hours, hasn't it?" she asked Dr. Peterson.

"God, yes. Closer to five."

The warm water poured down her leg. "Bob, you'll have to help me," Dr. Morris said. "I can't put enough pressure on this artery."

It was only then that it occurred to her that the warm water was blood.

"Whatever you do, don't move that leg! Hold perfectly still!" Dr. Peterson said.

It took thirty minutes to get the bleeding stopped. Both doctors looked tired.

"Can't you put a stitch in it?" she asked at one point.

"And risk two more holes in this?"

"I guess that does it," Dr. Morris said. "We'll get you cleaned up and into a fresh gown."

She was two-thirds onto the stretcher when a violent wave of nausea swept over her. Dr. Peterson jumped out of the way just in time.

"Oh!" she said. "How awful! I didn't have any warning."

"Don't think a thing about it," he said. "I'm in practice. I have a new baby. It's my own fault—I shouldn't have given you that water. We've never had anyone react to the dye *this* late."

There was a bright-red stain spreading over the front of her clean gown.

She hadn't been back in her room long when Dr. Jamison appeared. "I've been looking at your X-rays," he said. "You have an aneurysm of the left ventricle. That's a bulge—like a bulge you might have in an inner tube. It's still part of the heart wall, that is. The pictures aren't as clear as we'd like, but there's no doubt." He seemed terribly pleased. "I've asked Dr. Rudd to drop round to see you tomorrow."

"Is he a surgeon?"

"He is," Dr. Jamison said.

Dr. Lewis was excited, too. "I certainly gave my little talk last night to the wrong person," he said. "I've been laughing at the irony of it all afternoon. Dr. Allen's the one I should have given it to. I'm sorry."

"Have you seen the X-rays?" she asked.

"Yes, we've found the trouble."

"What does an aneurysm of the left ventricle mean?"

"Well, imagine a football, with one segment ballooned way out." He demonstrated with his hands. "The balloon is the aneurysm. It fills with extra blood, and the heart wears itself out trying to empty it. That's it, oversimplified."

"Did you know that Dr. Jamison is having a surgeon come see me tomorrow?"

"Dr. Rudd. There's a special thing about him. He's not only a very fine surgeon; he knows as much cardiology as any cardiologist. That's not generally true. Now we *really* have a team," he said with satisfaction. "Dr. Rudd, Dr. Jamison, and me."

"And me."

"Why, you're the most important member."

The intern who came round that night said, "I've been up to see your X-rays. All of us on the floor had a bet on what they'd show. I lost. I didn't think it was an aneurysm. I thought it was muscle failure."

"Did anyone win?"

"Yes. Dr. Jamison."

● ● ●

Dr. Rudd was in his surgeon's garb, a calm, avuncular-looking man, big enough to be imposing, with quick, amused eyes and a broad smile. He reminded her of someone. He shook her hand and sat on a chair beside the bed. "I've been studying your X-rays." He was carrying a used envelope, on the back of which he'd made a little drawing. "The heart looks like this." He held out the envelope. "Here's the aneurysm. Upstairs they estimate that it's thirty-seven per cent the size of the ventricle. I think it's larger—fifty, maybe. The pictures aren't very clear."

"Is that large?"

"Pretty large. Of course we don't know exactly. I hope we can get a better idea from the arteriogram. We've put you down for that for Friday morning." He spoke in a relaxed, Midwestern accent.

"Friday!"

"Providing you feel up to it."

"Dr. Rudd, what would the surgery be?"

"Well, you cut out the aneurysm and stitch the sides of the ventricular wall together. I'd also plan to take a vein from your leg and attach it to the aorta and run it across to the coronary artery, to give you a better blood supply. We've been doing that successfully."

"It sounds like a long operation."

"Oh, I'd say around six hours. Maybe a little longer."

"Do you think you're going to be able to do it?"

"Perhaps. We won't be sure until we have the arteriogram. Do you think you'll feel up to it Friday?"

"Of course."

"I'll be seeing you," he said.

A nurse she hadn't seen before came in next morning. "I'm Miss Josephson," she said. "Dr. Rudd's nurse. I've come to prepare you for your heart surgery."

"Physically or psychologically?"

Miss Josephson considered. "Psychologically, I guess. I work with all the open-heart surgery cases."

"But nothing's decided," she said. "They haven't even done the arteriogram."

"Dr. Rudd asked me to see you."

"I must be going to have it," she told Ellie that evening. "I had a visit from the psychological-preparation nurse."

● ● ●

The arteriogram took only an hour and a half. And only one catheter at a time, run up from the left femoral artery. It was done in a different department, by a different set of doctors. They used meticulous care and five variously sized catheters, whisking them in and out, to get pictures as sharp as they wanted. They had studied the catheterization X-rays. There was no trouble with the dye, no trouble with the artery.

She was scarcely downstairs again when Dr. Jamison appeared. "They got wonderful pictures," he said. "The aneurysm is bigger than we thought. But the really surprising thing is that the blood supply's so good. It explains your color. You don't look like a heart patient, you know. Practically no deposit on the arterial walls."

"*That's* good, isn't it?"

"It could hardly be better."

"We're set for surgery?"

"I don't see any reason why not."

They smiled at each other like a pair of conspirators.

● ● ●

Dr. Rudd came in the afternoon. In his hand was another used envelope, with another little drawing on the back. He sat down beside her. "There isn't any one man in the country who has made a specialty of this operation," he said, "but I'll be comfortable doing it if you would like to have me."

"I would," she said. "I've been hoping it would be possible."

"I have to tell you that we could get your chest opened up and I might decide the risk was too great to proceed. It's large. The men who did the arteriogram figure between fifty and sixty. They think nearer sixty. I still think fifty. It will depend on our judgment of the strength of what's left of the ventricle to carry on. Do you understand?"

"I understand."

"The blood supply's so good I shan't need to transplant the vein. That will cut the time down to four, four and a half hours. It takes an hour and a half just to open the chest."

"When can you do it?"

"We thought next Thursday, beginning around seven-thirty.

Tuesdays and Thursdays are my days. I could do it Wednesday, but you'd be fourth on the schedule. It will be best for you to be first. Dr. Jamison can be there. Dr. Lewis can arrange his hours to be there."

"That's almost a week. What do I do between now and then?"

"You stay right where you are. I don't want to lose this bed rest."

"As open-heart surgery goes," Dr. Lewis said, "this is moderate to large. There will be about a dozen doctors in the operating room—perhaps more. A lot of preliminary work's going on already—using the statistics from the X-ray studies to make graphs and charts that Dr. Rudd will need. Your back doctor has been over. He thinks your back should withstand things."

"Are you pleased?"

"Very." His eyes were bright. "It's what you want, isn't it?"

"You know it is."

● ● ●

After visiting hours that evening, an intern came into her room. He'd been drawing her blood every morning, but her only impression of him was of earnestness. "I see you've decided to have the surgery," he said.

Something in his tone made her say, "Don't you approve?"

"No, I don't. I don't think you know what you're doing. If you were my—"

"Mother?" she supplied.

"Well, yes. I wouldn't *let* you. You haven't any idea of the risk and the awful complications of this particular operation,

and I'm pretty sure no one has gone into them with you. I
don't think you even know what this surgery *involves*. Of
course I'm not the primary physician on the case."

"But Dr. Jamison approves."

"Dr. *Jamison*? Are you *sure*?"

"I thought I was."

"I'd suggest you talk it over with him tomorrow and *make*
sure." At the door he said again, "Of course I'm not the primary physician, but I felt I had to give you my opinion."

"Yes," she said. "Thank you. I'll talk to Dr. Jamison in the
morning." She kept her anger from showing, but she slept
very little that night.

"Dr. Jamison," she said, "I've been thinking. Are there particular risks and complications in this surgery I ought to know
about? Do you really approve of my having it?"

The expression of special pleasure that had been on Dr.
Jamison's face gave way to one of reserve. "Nobody's rushing
you into this," he said. "It's entirely your decision."

"That isn't what I mean. My decision was made before I
ever came in here. But I *would* like to know what the risk is."

"It makes no sense to talk about risks in a thing like this,"
Dr. Jamison said. "Risks are statistics. Averaging. So far as
you're concerned, they're one hundred per cent or they're zero."

"Dr. Rudd," she asked that afternoon, "what would you
say is the risk of this operation?"

Dr. Rudd reflected. "Oh, I'd say around thirty-five per cent
or a little more—something like that," he said comfortably.

"I don't know why I asked," she said to Ellie. "I'd take it
anything short of a hundred."

She told Dr. Lewis about the intern. He was indignant. "Why, that's one of the most bizarre things I've ever heard! Bizarre and inexcusable! Who was it?"

"I'm not going to tell you," she said. "I was furious, but I'm over it. He felt strongly and was acting on principle."

"I'm not against principle," Dr. Lewis said, "but he has to be told what to do with it. This is a teaching hospital. It would have been perfectly all right for him to bring his disapproval to me; we could have talked it over and I could have explained. To have come to you with it is inexcusable!"

Dr. Rudd and Dr. Jamison came in together the following morning. "All the residents and interns on the floor are upset about your surgery," Dr. Rudd said.

"Why?"

"They don't think you look sick enough." He laughed. "We've just had to tell them we know more than they do."

Dr. Jamison laughed, too. "I told your intern that if you were *my* mother I'd want you to have it," he said. "In fact, I'd be pushing you hard."

• • •

One evening, two doctors walking down the corridor stopped just beyond her door to discuss some changes in a patient's medication. One of them said in the saddest voice, "She's going to die, and she's such a nice woman."

"I could hear you saying something like that about me," she said to Dr. Lewis later. "And I wanted to tell you, if anything goes wrong, *don't grieve.*"

"I won't," he said.

"You can't always have your own way."

She had been moved across the hall to a room with sun and a river view. Her family came—her sister Beth, her dead brother's two daughters, whom she'd loved since they were babies and hadn't seen for a long time. The telephone rang, and there was the voice of her older niece. "I'm at Kennedy," she said. "I'll be right along." She was touched. Sometimes the young surprise you, she thought. They were all so pretty. The room was full of flowers. They sat together, the five of them, laughing and talking, and those days of waiting were like Christmas, before death, when the family was whole and had been together.

"There's always been enough love," she said to Dr. Lewis one night out of the blue. "I don't mean there haven't been disasters of love, and anguish, but there's always been some-one to whom you mattered enough and who mattered to you."

Curious. She was a private person, really—covered—but these days she was quite naked.

• • •

Dr. Rudd said, "I want to prepare you for the Intensive Care Unit. It can be a shock if you don't know what to ex-pect. It's an open room with four beds and a good deal of equipment. Bright lights are kept on twenty-four hours. You can't tell day from night. There's constant activity. You'll wake up with a large tube in your throat—not very comfort-able. It's connected to a machine that will be breathing for you. We'll get it out as soon as we can. There'll be a good many tubes. You'll be thirsty. We can't let you have anything to drink for a while. There'll be pain; we can't cover it entirely. You probably won't remember Thursday at all. After that, it depends."

"If I make it through surgery, am I safe?"

"No, the danger period lasts through the days in Intensive Care."

"I'm not afraid to die," she heard herself saying.

He made a dismissing gesture with his hand. "That's not the question," he said.

"Doesn't Dr. Rudd remind you of Father!" Beth said.

"That's it!" Ellie and she looked at each other in amazement. But she didn't tell him. It would have been too much.

Dr. Jamison prepared her for the Intensive Care Unit—"It's noisy. You won't get much sleep; just naps. Too much has to be done for you." And so did the psychological-preparation nurse, who came regularly to describe the world to which she would waken. "Everything of your own in this room will have to be taken away Wednesday," she said. "You can't have a thing with you except your toothbrush and a comb. There's no place to put it." A breathing machine was brought to her room on Monday, and Monday, Tuesday, and Wednesday the psychological-preparation nurse instructed her in its use and conducted breathing practice.

Wednesday, after lunch, the nurse in charge of the floor came into her room and announced formally, "As of four o'clock this afternoon, your name will be placed on the danger list."

• • •

"I'll see that you sleep tonight," Dr. Rudd told her. "They'll be getting you up early."

But she didn't. She was awake most of the night and glad to have a nurse come in at five-thirty. "One of the doctors from surgery will be down soon to put in your I.V. and a stomach tube," she said. She was a motherly woman, and she took her in her arms and cradled her for a moment. "You're very brave," she said. "We'll all be praying for you."

They came for her at seven—no hypodermic, no sedative—and upstairs they wheeled the stretcher into a small room adjacent to the operating room. There were doctors and nurses coming and going, all in surgical garb. They paid no attention to her but bustled about, obviously getting organized. Every now and then the door of the operating room opened and a blast of music poured out.

"Who's doing the anesthetic?" one of the nurses asked.

"Barnes," a doctor answered.

"Barnes!" someone said. Around the room eyebrows were raised and looks were exchanged.

"He's late. We're ready," the doctor said.

Almost as he spoke, a frowning, black-browed doctor strode into the room and over to her. "I'm Dr. Barnes," he said. "I'm going to put you to sleep."

There wasn't time to say a prayer. There wasn't time to count one.

$$+ + + 2$$

S HE CAME WHIRLING OUT OF A LONG TUNNEL AND
knew at once she was in the Intensive Care Unit. A wide
board was jammed across her throat. It kept her from asking
what time it was, and it seemed important to know. There
were people around her bed. Someone was calling her first name
loud. She was thirsty.

"Prick. This is your antibiotic," a woman's voice said.

"Prick. I'm giving you morphine."

Every time she opened her eyes, a nurse was bent over the
bed, doing something. She wore a blue uniform. It was always
the same nurse.

She felt splashed with ice water. "I'm going to turn on . . ."
Slowly, cold spread through her back and up into her head.
Her ears ached. Her teeth began to chatter.

"Prick." . . . "Prick."

There were other people in the room.

"I'm staying on an extra shift," her nurse said.

"But you can't," a doctor's voice said. "You'll be worn out."

"Please. Let's not argue. We're short."

There was something black dangling on her left wrist.

"Your sisters are here," the nurse said in the loud voice everyone said everything. "They're coming in for five minutes—
O.K?"

Ellie and Beth came toward her. They walked gingerly.
Their eyes looked frightened. They took her hand. "You're
beautiful," Beth said in her gentle voice. "Darling, you look
beautiful." That was what their mother had said when she
lay dying. In a hospital bed, a tiny, delicately boned woman,
with her head tipped up like a bird's. "Beth, you're beautiful,"
and to Beth's husband, who was dear to her, "John, you're
beautiful." "Mama, how about me?" she'd asked, teasing.
"Oh, *you!*" her mother had said with such tenderness it made
her eyes fill to remember. "Honey," Ellie said, "you're going
to be better soon"—the very words and loving tone she'd used
when they'd been made to leave the little dog they'd gone
together to the animal center to have put to sleep a few months
before. She would never get over not being allowed to stay
with him.

So she wasn't going to make it. Fact, not feeling. No feeling
at all.

"Everything is fine," Beth said.

She raised her eyebrows in denial.

"It is," Ellie said. "It really is. You're going to be all right."

"All three of your doctors told us so."

They both looked stricken.

"Do you know you're hitched up to a machine that costs
thirty-seven thousand five hundred dollars?" Ellie said. "It's
on loan. They're trying it out on you."

She pointed to her wrist, the one with the black marks,
wanting terribly to know the time.

"Do you want me to rub your arm?" Ellie asked. "I don't

think I dare. You have intravenouses going in both your hands."

She shook her head angrily.

They looked helpless.

She made an effort and traced the shape of her wristwatch. Those black marks were the dangling ends of sutures. What were they doing on her *wrist?*

"Oh," Ellie said. "You want to know the time. It's eleven-thirty."

Morning? Night? What day?

"I think that's enough," the nurse said.

"We'll be back tonight." They bent and kissed her.

What *day* was it?

● ● ●

The room was full of loud voices. "Joe! Joe! I'm going to . . ." "Lucy, you've *got* to. Now try harder. You can do it—O.K.?"

"I want you to take some deep breaths, O.K.?" the nurse said to her.

She was too thirsty, and the board in her throat hurt.

"Have you got the gases on her?" A man's voice.

"I'm just getting them." Her nurse.

Getting them where?

"Prick. I'm giving you morphine."

A little black woman in a bandanna turban came to the side of the bed and fell on her knees. "Oh, Jesus, Jesus!" She rocked back and forth. The nurse kicked her hard. "This is no place for praying," she said. "If you have to pray, find yourself some place where you aren't in the way. Get out!"

Had that little black woman really been there? "Hallucination?" her mind offered.

"I'm going to need more blood," her nurse said. "We're low. I ordered plenty."

"We had to use some for Joe," a doctor's voice said.

"But I ordered ten pints—more than enough. And we need more saline. I ordered plenty of that, too. Check with the clerk if you don't believe me."

"Joe's on it. Can't you use glucose?"

"I can't. Saline's what she's getting."

"Goddam it, and the weekend coming up!"

Dr. Rudd was at her right side. She couldn't open her eyes, but she recognized his voice. There were doctors on both sides of the bed. "This is the Novocain. . . ." That was all she heard him say.

The board in her throat was gone. She hadn't even felt them pull it out. But there was something dragging at her neck. It hurt in a different way; it was sore. She started to raise her hand toward it.

"You've had a tracheotomy," her nurse said, moving her hand back to her side. "There's a plastic tube there. Now you'll be able to breathe better."

Both her hands were strapped to boards.

They took out the plastic and put a thin tube down her throat and suctioned out the trachea. "Cough!" they said. "Cough!"

Dr. Jamison was there. "I know you're thirsty," he said.

"You're dehydrated. But we don't dare give you anything to drink. It might make you sick at your stomach, and then all hell could break loose."

Her nurse brought her a lollipop of cotton batting soaked in glycerine and lemon. It was cool on her lips and, briefly, in her mouth.

The doctors around the bed across from her were talking about Dr. Rudd. They were angry. "He's requiring so much care for"—she heard her name—"he's endangering the life of everyone else in this room," one of them said.

Dr. Rudd spoke up. "Please remember I'm the top man here," he said. "Any two-bit surgeon who can do a valvulotomy can have a patient in this unit. My operations are the big ones. So long as I have a patient here who needs care, she's going to get it." He was as calm as ever, but his voice was commanding.

What was he doing over there across the room?

"I'm turning on the thermal . . ." her nurse said. "We've got to get your fever down."

The cold. The earache. The chill. She shook all over.

Dr. Rudd was at her side. "That's not a normal chill," he said. "Get the heater."

All of a sudden she was warm.

There were doctors at the foot of the bed. It was dark. ". . . three five-per-cent strokes during the operation," one of them was saying. "They didn't tell you *that,* did they! Or what the tracheotomy has probably done to your vocal cords."

Oh God, she thought, she wasn't going to speak again!

Beth and Jean, their younger niece, came. Only two could come at one time. Ellie sent a letter. "I'll read it to you," Beth said. " 'Remember Liz Taylor had a tracheotomy and it didn't mar *her* beauty.' "

Now she could move her lips. "Glasses," she said, and she pointed to her eyes.

"Do your eyes hurt?" Beth asked.

She shook her head.

"Do you have a headache?"

"Never mind," she said with her lips.

"I think maybe she wants her glasses," Jean said.

"Oh, I feel so stupid!" Beth said. She went off, and after a while she and a nurse came back with the glasses and a tooth-brush and comb. They put the glasses on her, and at once the blur around her cleared. There was a big clock on the wall to the right.

"Would you like to write Ellie a note?" Beth asked.

She wrote dizzily at the bottom of Ellie's letter.

"We'll bring you something to write on tomorrow," Beth said, and they kissed her and went away.

The foot of another bed faced the foot of hers. A man was in it—Joe? Bottles and tubes were strung along both sides, and she could see the machine that was monitoring his heart. The line of the cardiogram jumped up and down. In the bed at her side, a cameo face in a frame of waved black hair lay on the pillow, unmoving. Lucy?

"I'm taking away the oxygen for a while," her nurse said. "I want you to take deep breaths—O.K.? I know it hurts, but you have to."

The nurse's name was spelled out in white stitching on her blue uniform: Carol.

"Have you got the gases?" an intern asked.

Nurses were arguing. A little blond nurse was saying, "But you could *show* me what to do. I'd be *glad* to work an extra shift. You can't manage as short as this."

"We'll manage," Carol said. "Betty's here and Dot's coming in."

"Please let me. I could take care of Joe for you. I'd ask about anything I wasn't familiar with."

"Will you kindly get the hell out of here?" one of the interns said. "Have you got the gases on her?"

"In a minute," Carol said.

"Prick." . . . "Prick."

"How are you going to feel"—it was her name the doctor was using—"to leave here knowing that three other people didn't make it because you got all the attention? How do you think you'll feel *then*?"

Whenever Dr. Rudd came into the room, everything grew calm. He was talking across the bed to Carol. He bent over and lifted two large tubes. They were full of pink fluid. "*These* aren't doing any good," he said. "They might as well come out. This is going to hurt."

"Look at me! Look at me!" Carol said, and she turned her head. It felt as if half her side had given way.

Where had those tubes been, she wondered.

"Dr. Rudd tells me the arterial line and both drains from the heart are out," Dr. Lewis said.

Arterial line?

Lucy was leaving. She had summoned her doctor from Westchester and demanded to be removed to another hospital where she would be properly looked after. There she sat in a wheel chair next to her bed, in a brown flannel suit and a beige satin blouse with French cuffs. "I'll sign you out," her doctor said, "but it is entirely on your own responsibility. I warn you, it's a matter of life and death."

Then Lucy was gone. Then she was back, still in her wheel chair, in her brown suit and fine beige blouse. But when she looked again there was the cameo face, unmoving, on the pillow.

"We're going to get you into a more comfortable bed," Carol said. "You're still in the cardiac bed you came from the operating room in. Don't move—we'll do it."

A great gash above her groin at the left was pulled together with a long line of sutures. No one had prepared her for *that*.

Carol brought her a tray and started to feed her. Jello. Ginger ale. Custard. She turned her head away.

"Dr. Rudd wants you to eat," Carol said.

She turned her head, in a rage that the food was all sweet.

She heard her name from across the room. ". . . may make it or she may not, but Dave Rudd will get a brilliant article out of this, either way." So that was his first name: David.

May make it?

She opened her eyes. She wrote on her pad, "Do you know I can hear?"

Carol gave her a speculative look. "Yes," she said.

The intern in charge came into the room. He came over to her bed. "You're some spring chicken, *you* are!" he said. He had not spoken to her before.

Except from the people taking care of her, she heard her name only one more time. Out of blackness, a Chinese voice called to her. "This is the year of the lion," the voice said. "And *you* are a lion and will fight your way through."

Joe's cardiogram was a straight line. A crowd of doctors surrounded him. They were wheeling his bed toward the door. But when she next woke up there he was as before. Another hallucination? Only they no longer called him Joe. They called him Sam, Tom, Jim, Hank—any old name—and Carol went to spend her time with him.

"Is that Joe?" she wrote.

The nurse said yes.

• • •

All the pricks now were antibiotics. There was no more morphine.

Dr. Rudd said, "I've asked Dr. Williams to come in to see you. He's a lung specialist. He'll be in sometime this morning."

Dr. Williams brought another doctor with him. They were there for almost two hours. They sat her up carefully; they laid her down. "She should be having thirty-five-per-cent pure oxygen," Dr. Williams said to the intern. "There are air pockets. I want her waked up every hour and pounded on the back, then suctioned out. I'll go write the orders. We'll be in tomorrow. We'll need more X-rays and cultures."

They took blood three and four times a day, and when they couldn't get it from her veins they took it for the cultures from her bruised right femoral artery. Both hands had swollen monstrously from the intravenous, and the needles were removed; her hands were wrapped in hot vaseline packs.

"Are you coughing enough?" Dr. Jamison asked. "Here." He lifted her up. He put his hands on either side of her rib cage. "Take a deep breath. That's good. Now cough for me. I'll hold you. You're going to have to bring up whatever this is."

She felt as if she were split asunder, and it was choking with the plastic tube in her throat.

"Again."

"I've asked Dr. Ellis from the Infectious Diseases Department to come see you," Dr. Rudd said. "We have to track down the cause of your fever."

Next morning Dr. Ellis came with two members of his staff. *They* sat her up carefully; they laid her down. Dr. Ellis had piercing blue eyes that looked at her with sympathy. "Do you hurt anywhere?" he asked.

Good God, she thought.

"We'll want cultures," Dr. Ellis said.

"When can I drink?" she wrote on her pad for Dr. Jamison. "You should be drinking now," he said. "Just not too much at one time." He turned to the nurse. "Get her some ginger ale."

The nurse brought an icy bottle of Schweppes ginger ale. She poured it into a tall paper cup and bent a straw and gave it to her. "Not too fast," she said, but she let her drink the whole thing. "Good?"

The fever was like a little tent. The chill, then warmth settled over her—a shelter—and she dozed. But the hypothermic blanket made her ears ache and brought on a chill of a different nature. She dreaded it, though the suctioning was worse. "Take a deep breath," they said. "Now cough!"

One night the intern who was on thirty-six-hour duty reeled into the room from wherever it was he'd been sleeping. "My God, what's the matter *now!*" he shouted.

● ● ●

Lucy had left and three people had come and gone from the bed across from where Lucy's bed had been when Dr. Rudd said, "Dr. Jamison thinks you would do better in another room, where the lights are out at night and you'd get more sleep and privacy. There's no place free where I'd want to put you today, but maybe tomorrow."

The next unit was across the hall, just beyond the nurses' station. There were four beds in this room, too, but more space between and a chair for each bed. There was less machinery. A familiar profile lay on the pillow to her left. It was Lucy. But that afternoon Lucy was wheeled out in her bed and someone else was wheeled in.

She was off the monitor, though there was a tank of oxygen with a breathing attachment at one side of her bed, and a moisture-making machine with a mask that was kept on her face most of the time; there was medicine in it. The suctioning equipment was at the head of the bed. A bell was pinned within reach of her hand. Nurses were not in this room all the time. They came in, one for each patient, several times a day and at night. Voices were quieter. The other patients in the room could talk to one another. Visitors were permitted to stay longer. Tension was lower.

She sat on the edge of the bed and dangled her legs over the side, and the second day she was helped into a chair, where she stayed for a few minutes. That afternoon a small basket of flowers was brought in to her. Dozens of roses—cream and yellow and light pink and deep. The handle was twined with pale-blue velvet, and babies'-breath made a delicate veiling all the way round. The nurse put the basket on the window sill beside her bed, a gentle thing to look at after these ungentle days.

It was in this room that she began to write, "I can't get enough air." Pain burned from armpit to armpit through to her back. There was no relief from it, and one night she remembered a story about a simple-minded black woman who came home to find her mother dead; she couldn't move for the terror of it, and she dropped to her knees and repeated over and over, "Bless God, bless God" until she had enough space in her head to accept what she must.

"Bless God," she said, "bless God, bless God, bless God, bless God . . ."

Dr. Rudd seemed to know how she felt without her telling him. "Nothing short of Demerol or morphine will do you any good," he said, "and we can't risk them for fear of depressing your breathing."

That night such a tearing pain came with a fit of coughing that the nurse called a doctor, and he called an X-ray technician, who came at once and took an X-ray of her chest. In the middle of the night.

"There's fluid in your lungs," Dr. Rudd said. "I want better X-rays than we can get here," and she was wheeled down to the X-ray Department. As she was waiting to be wheeled back, Dr. Rudd came toward her. "I want a look at those X-rays," he said as he went by.

"A section of lung has collapsed," he told her up in the room. "You're going to have to cough more. Don't be afraid. I have you put together so tightly you couldn't come apart if you tried."

"It feels like my idea of pleurisy *and* pneumonia," she wrote to Ellie, "but of course I've never had either."

When she coughed, Ellie held her.

They did the suctioning oftener. Dr. Rudd did it every time he came in, and he washed the plastic tube himself and replaced it. He was more skillful than the nurses; it was less strangling.

When night came and the lights were out, a nurse helped her sit up with her legs over the side of the bed and she put her head on the bedside table and recited "Bless God" endlessly—a litany to help endure what seemed unendurable. She dreamed that one of the doctors came and with his own hands gave her a hypodermic and a respite. She dreamed of a beaded glass of Schrafft's lemonade, with a sprig of mint showing cool over the rim. Fluids were restricted once more.

One night a nurse spent most of the night with her, working around the bed to make her comfortable. That night she slept. The morning after, the woman in the bed next her asked to be moved from the room. "I can't get well beside anyone as sick as *she* is," she said. They wheeled her out as soon as lunch was over.

"We've decided to take off some of that fluid," Dr. Rudd told her, and in the afternoon two interns came in with a trolleyful of equipment and bent her over her bedside table.

"Get a resident!" the first intern called in a loud, urgent voice when he saw the fluid flowing into the bottle. "Don't look!" But she looked anyway. It was red.

The resident was there with two other doctors in seconds. "It's all right," the resident said in an authoritative voice, and in a different voice to one of the interns with him, "Quick! Run this over to the centrifuge!" In his first voice he said to the intern with the needle, "I wouldn't take off more than two hundred c.c.'s."

When the job was finished, they all moved off, but the second intern—he had a round, jolly face—came back and wrote on her pad, "Bye Bye."

"This has nothing to do with your *heart*," Dr. Lewis said. "So far as your *heart* goes, everything is right on schedule." He had brought her two new pads and two new pencils with fresh, sharp points.

Beth brought lengths of heavy yarn, and she or Ellie brushed her hair straight up onto the top of her head and tied it there with a small, bright bow. She couldn't lift her arms to brush her hair for herself.

Dr. Jamison said, "Things couldn't be better, especially now that you have your hair combed."

"I think they think I'm depressed," she wrote to Ellie. "They're all trying to cheer me up."

"Are you?" Ellie asked.

"No, I just can't get enough air."

● ● ●

An older surgeon on the staff—Dr. Hollister—came along with the interns on morning rounds and took the dressing off her incision. He poked and prodded. "You have an abscess under a stitch here," he said. "I'll leave it for Dr. Rudd."

Dr. Rudd appeared shortly. "This may be what we've been looking for," he said, almost with satisfaction. "The cause of your fever. I'm going to have to open it up. We'll get a culture on it and see." He opened it up at once—a long stretch in the middle of the incision. He came twice a day and irrigated and packed and dressed the opening. It looked like a piece of raw steak, and when she coughed, air whistled through it. "I want you to lie on your left side and cough for ten minutes every two hours," Dr. Rudd said. "I don't want to put a drain in unless I have to."

"I can't lie on my left side," she wrote.

"Can you lie across your bedside table? That would be all right."

"I don't think it's a serious infection," Dr. Jamison said. "You look too good."

"Your fever's up but the white count is not," Dr. Rudd said. "I'm not going to put in a drain."

"You're having some bad luck," Dr. Lewis said. "It will end."

● ● ●

But she was making progress. Every day she was helped into a chair, and one morning she walked drunkenly across the hall to the washroom. She dipped her washcloth in water the nurse had drawn and lifted it halfway to her face. The face in the mirror was a travesty of her own—thin, mostly eyes and cracked, encrusted lips. She looked at it briefly. Then she sat on the toilet seat and rang the bell to be helped back to her bed. That day she didn't get washed at all. The nurses urged her to walk, to cough, to eat more.

"I can't," she wrote to the last. "I can't swallow this food." It was dreadfully cooked—a soft diet, gray, and without any seasoning at all.

Ten days after he had put it in, Dr. Rudd took the plastic tube out of her trachea. "I think things are healed enough now, and I know you'll be more comfortable."

She could speak at once, her voice not quite natural but her own.

"Listen!" she said to Beth that afternoon.

"Listen!" she said to Ellie. "I can *talk!*"

There were two more areas of fluid in her lungs. "We can't isolate anything of significance," the Infectious-Diseases doctor said. "You've had too many antibiotics." The doctors debated drawing it off. One day they thought they would; the next day they thought they would wait.

"One thing I *couldn't* stand—to go back to the operating room," she said to Dr. Lewis.

"There is no thought of *that*," he said sternly.

"I haven't any margin left."

• • •

Now that she had her voice, she told Dr. Rudd what she had heard in Intensive Care.

He sat down to talk. "It sounds to me like a bad trip," he said. "Anesthesia today is very sophisticated, and you had a fever of a hundred and four and a lot of morphine those days. No one in the world would have said that kind of thing to you —it's unthinkable. It was hallucination."

"Some of it," she said. "I even thought that at the time. But I'd bet you on a good part of what I heard. My mind was in order."

"Perhaps you don't know that I'm in charge of the Intensive Care Unit. I'm in there a lot. The tension you felt was all from the patients—not the staff. I would know."

"But it's not there when you are. You bring quiet with you. I think you haven't any idea."

"It was hallucination," he said in a kind voice. "And no wonder. I wasn't anywhere near the room that time you heard me defending myself."

"Then someone must have spoken up for you."

He shook his head. "And I never do an article on just one case."

The next day, Dr. Rudd sat down beside her again. "I've

been talking to Dr. Hollister about your experience. He says there were things said that you could have misunderstood. I haven't got hold of Carol yet, and I want to talk to some of the others."

Dr. Lewis said, "It had to have been a bad trip. Dr. Rudd told me about it and that was my first thought, too."

"Not all of it," she said stubbornly.

"It doesn't make sense. There's no such thing as a five-percent stroke."

She told Beth and Ellie. "I'll accept that Dr. Rudd wasn't in the room when I thought I heard him, and I know that little black woman was hallucination—I knew it at the time. And that Lucy couldn't possibly be out of bed and in a wheel chair—"

"But she was," Ellie said. "We had to climb over that wheel chair out in the hall when we came to see you Sunday."

"Did she have on a brown suit?"

"I didn't notice the color," Beth said, "but she did have on a suit and a beige satin blouse."

Two weeks after surgery, she was moved to a third room in the unit—the one farthest from the nurses' station. Four beds, but the people in them were less sick. The oxygen went with her, and the moisture-making machine; the suctioning was over. She was walking rather shakily in the corridor, where there was a rail to hang on to. And still the examinations, the X-rays; still the blood tests.

After four days, Dr. Rudd said, "Wouldn't you be happier out of here and in a private room? I have one for you. Admissions said there wasn't a thing available, but I talked to the administrator, and when I called Admissions again it seems there had been one all along. A mystery. The food up there is better—a different food service. We want to get you eating."

She was smiling so widely when Dr. Jamison arrived that he said, "Well, I see you've heard the news. This afternoon. I'm going to shift you to a freer diet. You can have some salt. In fact, except for a moderate sodium restriction, you can have anything you want." He went through his usual examination. "You still have that fluid and a collapsed wedge," he said. "And fever. We'd like to get rid of them."

● ● ●

The new room was large, with the most beautiful view of the river she had ever seen. And perfectly broiled lamb chops for dinner, with a linen napkin and a nicely appointed tray. She ate almost half the food.

"That's better," Dr. Lewis said.

"You're going to have to cough more!" Dr. Rudd said. "Take a deep breath. *Cough!*" He patted her on the back as if she were a baby.

There was a large armchair to sit in by the window, and her own bathroom, though they didn't let her use it yet. Here she was not expected to wash herself but was given a bath in bed. She began to feel clean.

"I'm aware of those wires you've got me put together with," she said on an uncomfortable day to Dr. Rudd.

"No wires," he said. "You're much too thin. I used a very strong grade of Orlon."

He was still dressing the opened-up incision, and one morning he worked on it with forceps. The next afternoon the pain across her chest from armpit to armpit was beyond bearing, and tears began to roll down her face in a freshet. Just tears. It was the first time she had cried. She couldn't stop, even when Dr. Lewis came at dinnertime. "I seem to have lost my composure," she said, "and I can't get it back. I've hurt too long."

He left the room. "One of the nurses will bring you something in a minute," he said when he came back, and he stood by her bed and put the teabag on her tray into the pot of hot water and poured her out a cup of tea. "Drink this," he said. "Do you like anything in it?" He waited with her until she had taken the capsule the nurse brought in and was easier.

From then on, she got Darvon on a regular schedule, and when her fever went over a hundred and one, two Tylenol. She welcomed the fever.

• • •

"I'm going to start pushing you," Dr. Jamison said. "I want you out in the hall walking. A nurse will take you."

That afternoon she walked half the length of the hall and back, and the next day she walked the full length. The third day she walked twice, and she walked Ellie to the elevator when she left at the end of visiting hours. "I've got to get out of here," she said.

In the night, she felt the rhythm of her heart change. Dr. Lewis came early in the afternoon. It was Thursday, and he was going away for a long weekend. He listened to her chest.

He went out and a few minutes later brought in a cardiograph machine. Moving unhurriedly, without speaking, he took a cardiogram. He studied the strips.

"It's different, isn't it," she said. "I felt it happen."

"Did you tell anyone?"

"No, I didn't want any more fussing."

He went out again and came in with tubes and a hypodermic. He took the blood as silently as he had done the cardiogram, and he put the tubes and the strips in his pocket. "I'll turn these over to Dr. Jamison," he said. "See you Monday. Maybe Sunday evening."

Dr. Jamison came first thing Friday. He listened to her heart. He stood at the foot of the bed, looking down at her appraisingly. "I'm going to move you," he said. "There's a change, and while it may not be serious, it's potentially dangerous. I want you in Coronary Care. Our nurses know what they're doing; they can read cardiograms. I'll go make arrangements."

He was back shortly. "All set," he said. "They'll be right up for you."

"I can't just go in a wheel chair?"

"No. Wouldn't you like me to call your sister? It might be a shock for her to come to this room and find you gone. If you'll give me her number, I'll do it after we have you settled in." He looked around the room. "You won't be able to take your flowers," he said. "I'm sorry."

Dr. Jamison stayed with her. A nurse came in to pack. "It's the best coronary-care unit in the world," he said. "I set it up myself. I'd better prepare you: we treat every patient who comes in as if he'd had a heart attack. I don't think you have, but I can't be sure until we run some tests, and I'm not taking any chances. We keep you on a monitor, of course, and under constant surveillance. It will be safer to have you there over the weekend."

"Just over the weekend?"

"That's all I anticipate."

A procession moved into the room: two aides trundling a narrow bed and an attractive, purposeful nurse pushing a monitor. Dr. Jamison introduced her. "And this is our battery-powered monitor," he said. "We use a different method for connecting the leads from anything you've had—needles in the arms and thighs. We get a better contact, and they don't slip out."

The nurse put the needles in deftly. Her manner was professionally reassuring. "There, that's not so bad, now, is it?" She spoke in a French-Swiss accent. "And I've brought you an intravenous gown. It makes things easier with the wires and tubing. Now we'll get you onto our cardiac bed. I warn you, it's hard!"

She started to move herself toward the bed.

"Don't move!" Dr. Jamison said. "I don't want you moving a muscle!" He came over and took one corner of the sheet she was lying on, the nurse took one, and on the opposite side each of the aides took one; she was transported to the narrow, hard bed without a breath of effort.

Miss Townsend, the head nurse on the floor, came after her as she rolled down the corridor. "You'll be coming back to us, dear," she said. "Don't think you won't! We'll save your room for you."

They almost filled the elevator. She turned her head away from the curious eyes of the other passengers, embarrassed.

3

ORONARY CARE WAS ON A LOWER FLOOR. SHE WAS wheeled into a little room right at the center of the station, where duplicates of all the monitors traced cardiograms and blinked their red lights on and off. The outer wall had two large windows, and, except for the door, the wall facing the station was entirely windowed. The curtains around those windows and the bed were bittersweet. The little room was freshly painted; everything was immaculate.

"I'll be back in a few minutes," Dr. Jamison said, and he left her to the nurse and aides, who shifted her wires to a monitor on the wall behind her bed.

An intern came in and started an intravenous at the bend of her right arm. "I hate to put one here—you have to be careful not to bend your arm; the needle could break—and I hate to immobilize your right hand," he said. "But you haven't got another vein that's worth a damn. They've all collapsed."

"But why an I.V.?"

"Everyone has an I.V. for as long as he's in Coronary Care. We use it for medication. It can make as much as ten minutes' difference in an emergency."

"We want you on oxygen for your first twenty-four hours," the nurse said, and she clipped rubber tubing into her nostrils.

48

"And since you have a fever we'll just turn on the air-conditioning. Why don't you try to get a little rest? We'll be bothering you enough!"

On the wall behind her, red lights went on and off with a sharp ping-ping-ping, and the cardiogram traced its way noiselessly across the screen.

Dr. Jamison was in again. "I'm starting you on something that should take care of that arrhythmia," he said. "We'll be giving it to you in toxic dose, so speak up if you have any reaction. And don't worry! You're in good hands."

Dr. Rudd came in the afternoon. *He* stood at the foot of the bed, looking down at her appraisingly. "We are mystified but not alarmed," he said.

"Was it the walking?"

"I hope not."

Ellie came after work. "Do you know I can only stay for five minutes? And you can only have immediate family? Five minutes out of an hour. That means Jean and me, unless we ring in Sarah as a sister. She has time and would like to come. Jean can't make it every afternoon."

"Yes," she said, "I'd like that. Did Dr. Jamison call you?"

"Almost scared me to death, but I suppose it would have been worse if he hadn't."

"I can't have any flowers."

"Did you remember that this is Good Friday? Sunday's Easter."

"Your time's up," a nurse said at the door.

● ● ●

In Coronary Care, they took blood more often and in larger quantities than they had anywhere else she had been. Some days four and five times; sometimes even in the night. Her veins got harder and harder to get blood from. "But why?" she protested. "I've been tested and tested."

"You're still running a fever, and there's still fluid in your lungs. We have to keep trying to find the cause. It might be something we could cure."

"I'm thirsty," she said often.

"I'm sorry, you're on restricted fluids. We can't let you have anything more to drink."

The food was like the food in Intensive Care. She couldn't eat, though aides offered to feed her and were careful to cut up her meat and butter her bread.

On Easter Sunday, Ellie brought a large shopping bag. She took out the dear basket that had held the roses, and a bunch of tiny, bright-yellow chrysanthemums and a big bunch of wide white daisies. "They can throw them out tomorrow if they want to," she said. "You're going to have flowers for Easter!" She put the basket on top of the air-conditioner, and she took out a large bunch of little white grapes and washed them and put them on a table next the bed in a bowl she had brought. "From South America, not from California. You can eat them in the night. They might keep you from getting so thirsty. I'll rub your back before I go. Wouldn't you like your hair brushed?"

Monday morning Dr. Jamison said cheerfully, "Well, we haven't made it on our first try; I'm shifting to another drug," and he told her what it was.

"No change?"

"No change. Yet. Don't worry, we'll get it."

"How long do you figure it's going to take?"

"Oh, just a few more days. Give us to Wednesday. Remember, this is in toxic dose, too. Let us know."

"This is Dr. Jamison's party," Dr. Rudd said, but he came every day and changed the dressing, and he explained with care that he was going away for ten days, and the date he would be back. "I get into town on Sunday," he said, "and I want to find you out of here."

"If the beat doesn't get corrected?"

"You can live with it. It's regularized now—a bigeminy beat, pretty steady. It just means a less efficient heart. I'd rather it got corrected."

The second drug made her sick at her stomach, and Dr. Jamison stopped it and substituted a third. Then he combined two. That made her sick, and he tried a fifth. "Give us till Friday," he said. "That will just be a week. You're stubborn."

"Dr. Jamison doesn't like to be thwarted," one of the interns said.

Once more, pain from her chest settled through into her back. When she woke up in the night she was unable to move and had to ring for help.

"What position do you want to be in?" the nurse or aide would ask.

"I don't know. I hurt so much I can't imagine being comfortable."

They were kind. They brought extra pillows. "Well, let's try this," and sometimes it helped, but night after night, except for brief periods, she lay reciting "Bless God bless God bless God bless God" until she numbed her mind to feeling, or morning came.

The Infectious-Diseases doctor began to bring her paperback mysteries, and though her eyes slid away from the print, she read them, one after another. She read them all day and into the night, but slowly.

"I don't mean to be ungrateful," she said to Dr. Jamison on Thursday, "but I'm not sure I can stand it here much longer. I think it's partly being tied down."

"No need to apologize. The normal tolerance for this unit is six days; a good many psychological studies have been made of it. We'll get you up into a chair for a bit. That ought to help."

Interns and nurses came in during the night. "Your blood pressure's dropped," a nurse said one night, and she brought in an intern and they took her blood pressure over and over. "I can't even get it," he said. "I'll ask the resident to come in. We'd better give you some oxygen."

With that, all her holds seemed precarious.

● ● ●

Friday morning Dr. Jamison said, "Do you think you could endure it till Monday? I want to try something entirely different: Dilantin. It's been used for years for epilepsy. About two years ago we found that it had an effect on heart rhythm. I'll be starting you on such a large dose I'll have to have you here. It wouldn't be safe. Monday is a fast promise."

"Whether it's corrected or not?"

"Whether it's corrected or not."

What could she say? But when a new intern came in to shift the intravenous and thrust his long, broad needle into her painful veins in ten different places without finding a place to let it rest, she cried. It was like the earlier time—all tears —and, like the earlier time, she couldn't stop. "I can't let you do it again," she said finally. "I don't care."

"Why?" she asked the nurse who came in as he left. *"Why* wouldn't he get someone else? *Why* would he keep trying?"

"Ego," the nurse said. "It's his damn ego. He wouldn't admit he couldn't do it. I can't *stand* it when they hurt the patients. Here, let me wash your face. I'll get you Dr. Kay. He's considered the best intern in the whole hospital."

The tears were still falling into her pillow when Dr. Kay came in. He didn't say a word, but he got the needle into a vein on the very first try and it scarcely hurt.

"You know that intern felt as bad as you did about what happened," Dr. Lewis said in the afternoon. "He was just telling me about it."

"Then why didn't he go get someone who knew what he was doing!" she said in an ugly voice.

Dr. Lewis looked shocked.

Around dinnertime Dr. Jamison stopped in. "Is there anything we could do to make things more bearable for you?" he asked. "Would it help if you could have more company and they could stay longer?"

"It might."

"I'll arrange it. The rule's adamant and the nurses won't like it, but if they say anything tell them to get in touch with me. I'll leave word with the clerk. Have your sister stay with you a while when she comes this evening. And over the week-end."

"I'm so ashamed," she said. "But I feel like an animal in a trap."

"There's no reason to be ashamed," he said.

Saturday, she walked twenty-five feet or so down the corridor outside her room. The procedure was elaborate. The battery-powered monitor was wheeled in, her wires were connected to it, two freshly filled hypodermics were placed on top ("Are those for an emergency?" she asked the nurse. "That's right"), the intravenous bottle was transferred to a pole on wheels. An aide supported her and pushed the intravenous pole; another aide pushed the monitor; the nurse walked backward, reading the cardiogram. "It's regular!" she called. "She's out of the bigeminy." The interns at the desk came to look and walk backward with the nurse. It was like a parade.

In bed again, wired to her own monitor, her heart returned to its irregular pattern.

"I guess we need to keep you on your feet," Dr. Jamison said.

Sunday, two interns stuck their heads in her door. She braced herself.

"We've come to check up on you," one of them said.

"Dr. Bye Bye!" She held out her left hand.

They gave her the news of the Intensive Care Unit. "You were there for Joe's cardiac arrest, weren't you?" one of them asked.

"Was that why he was wheeled out of the room?"

"Yes, we had to take him to the O.R."

"His mind was gone after that, wasn't it?"

"Yes."

"Did he make it?"

"No, poor devil, but it was just as well."

"I thought I imagined it."

"No."

"Remember when you took off the fluid and hollered for the resident? I knew that wasn't blood."

"If you did, you knew more than we did. You should have seen the resident's face—it was ashen. We thought I was in your liver."

"I'm going to get out of here tomorrow," she told them.

● ● ●

Dr. Jamison was late coming in Monday morning. "I have bad news for you," he said. "There isn't a room available, not in the section you want, where the food's good. I've just been over to Admissions. They will have one tomorrow on your old floor. Miss Townsend said she'd hold it for you. I'm terribly sorry but there isn't a thing I can do."

She nodded, but she had no defenses left. She told everyone who came into her room that she was desperate.

The nurse who brought her medication on Tuesday morning smiled and said, "Well, we're all set for eleven o'clock," and the nurse's aide who bathed her said, "I guess we'd better get *you* cleaned up early."

Eleven o'clock came, and twelve, and one, and two, and finally the head nurse came in and said, "They've given that

room to another patient. Admissions wouldn't let Miss Townsend hold it. She tried. There isn't anything else. But there
will be tomorrow on another floor."

"I don't know if they told you how upset everyone was," Dr.
Lewis said. "Dr. Jamison went to Admissions. *I* went to Admissions. Interns called. Nurses called. Tomorrow *is* sure. I've
checked myself with both Admissions and the head nurse on
the floor. Tomorrow will come."

"I know," she said. "And I know I'm acting like a child. But
I feel as if I shall *die* if I don't get out of here."

"Twelve days is a long time to be in this unit."

"The rhythm isn't any different, is it."

"It has very brief periods of being normal, but no, not
really. You can live with it, you know. It isn't something you
can't live with."

● ● ●

She had been in her new room only an hour or so when
the rhythm of her heart shifted back to normal. Dr. Jamison
could hear it. The cardiogram he ordered showed the change.

"Was it the Dilantin?" she asked him.

"No. *You* did it." He sounded half disgusted. "I'm going
to keep you on it, though, just as a precaution." He was leaving
that evening for the rest of the week, for meetings in the
Middle West. "I've ordered some iron for you," he said. "We've
taken so much blood your hemoglobin's dropped. You'll have
to be on it for a few months. And you can go back to a regular
diet. We want you to eat."

"Are we on our own for the rest of the week?" she asked Dr. Lewis at dinnertime.

"It looks that way. And the intern who'll be looking after you isn't an activist. I've just been talking to him. Nothing but blood for pro time and potassium. I want you to rest."

Three benign days. The fever was lower; X-rays showed that the fluid in her lungs was less; the opened incision was definitely filling in. When she coughed, the air no longer whistled through it.

One evening, the intern from the very first floor she'd been on, the one who had disapproved of her surgery, came up to see her. "I'm so glad you're all right," he said, and he sat on the edge of the bed and held her hand and he didn't say another thing.

Dr. Rudd walked into her room Sunday afternoon. She took his hand in both of hers, and after a few seconds he brought his left hand up and covered hers. "I've missed you," she said. "Dr. Rudd, why do you suppose I minded the Coronary Care Unit so much more than Intensive Care?"

"Because you were more alert." He smiled. "If you stay here much longer, you may be the first patient I've ever discharged to go back to work the next day."

• • •

"How much longer do you think it will be?" she asked Dr. Lewis.

"Oh, the day will come when all four of us agree that you're ready. A week or two, I'd think. You have to be stronger than you are."

"You've lost seven pounds," Dr. Rudd said. "Try to eat more."

"You've got some premature beats still," Dr. Jamison said. "But we aren't going to hold you up for those. They'll go away in time, we hope. And we won't hold you up for your fever; it's coming down. You'll probably have it for a few weeks after you get home. I'll want you to take your temperature regularly."

"Did you ever decide what caused it?"

"We never did."

"Or the arrhythmia?"

"That, either."

She was sitting up in a chair. With help, she was walking to the sun room. She was restless. "Isn't it time?" she asked Dr. Lewis.

"Not quite. Soon."

One morning Dr. Rudd said, "Whenever the other two agree it's all right, it's all right with me. I want a last cardiogram taken at rest and immediately after walking, and a chest X-ray, and that will do it so far as I'm concerned."

"I feel you've given me back my life," she said. It was something she'd been wanting to say to him. "How does it feel to give a person her life?"

Dr. Rudd made his dismissing gesture. "I don't think in those terms," he said. "I'm a surgeon. Surgeons are doers."

"I think you're ready," Dr. Jamison said. "It's going to take six months, you know—possibly a year—to reach your maximum level. Don't get discouraged. Remember you're not sixteen. I'll want to see you in two weeks' time. You've been a wonderful patient—we couldn't have asked for more." He gave her an affectionate pat.

"How about Saturday morning?" Dr. Lewis said. "Would you like that? It would only be a few days longer in any case, and why be here over the weekend. I can come down to see you. I think you'll get better faster at home."

MONTHS LATER, BACK AT WORK AND BEGINNING to be active again, she was in Dr. Lewis's office.

"You're well," he said. "Oh, it will be some months yet, but I don't have to worry about you any more."

A question had turned up in her mind. "How many of those operations have they done?" she asked.

"Between fifteen and twenty—seventeen is the exact number, I believe."

Dr. Rudd had said the risk was thirty-five per cent or a little more. She figured. Had they lost six? Seven?

"I ran into Dr. Rudd in the corridor today," Dr. Lewis said. "We stopped and congratulated ourselves."

"You mean I'm a credit to us?"

"To us and a good many others you don't know anything about." His expression was thoughtful—entirely serious.

They sat for a moment, unsmiling, looking at each other. Oh God, she thought, those nightmare days. Dear God, the miracle.